DELDRIC DUNNING

Running to Better Health

10 Ways Running Has Changed My Outlook On Life

Contents

1

Introduction

Running for me was a new experience. I mean, I was always very athletic, playing football and basketball growing up. However, I never ran for the love of it. To be quite honest, I hated it! I could barely run five laps around the basketball court without stopping to gasp for air. Two things I will never forget during my high school days were those suicides we did for basketball practice and those 40-yard sprints we did during football practice. If someone had told me to run a mile during that time, I would have looked at them as if they were crazy! Throughout my high school and college days, I managed to stay around 160-175 lbs. For the most part, during that time in my life, I considered myself a strong yet skinny guy. As I finally moved on and entered the business world, things like going to P.E. class and going to practice for basketball and football were all things of the past. I didn't have anyone to tell me when to work out anymore.

After nearly five years in the business world, I gradually started to put on the pounds without notice. I never worried too much since I had a relatively fast metabolism, eating whatever I wanted. In 2015, I decided to run my very first 5K (roughly 3.2 miles), which was sponsored by the company I worked for back then. I begin to train myself by taking baby steps. At that time, I could not run a full mile without stopping. I would run half and then walk half. It was tough, but it was the first time in a long time I challenged myself physically. When it finally came time for the race, I felt I was very prepared. Boy, was I mistaken! I felt like crap at the end of that race. My legs were sore, my chest burning, and I hardly could catch my breath. It took me roughly 35:00 minutes to complete. That race reminded me why I hated running in the first place. I said to myself that I would never try that again. A year later, our company sponsored another 5K run called Run For Kenya, in which the proceeds raised from this race were used to help operate and maintain a brand-new medical and dental clinic in Meto, Kenya. So, I decided to do it for the cause and trained once more. My time was slightly better but felt the same as the last race. After that race, I said I was done with running for good! I ended up ballooning to over 230 lbs, which was the heaviest I had ever been.

As time passed, I realized how precious our time is here on Earth. I started getting hit with some very tragic losses within my family, as well as friends that I was very close with, some of whom were pretty young. Traumatized by the thought of death quite a bit, I started to suffer from a lot of anxiety. I did not have any way of coping with it at the time, so I just dealt with it the best way I knew how. I later found a new job and relocated for a fresh start. Still unhappy with how I looked or felt, I started working out at the local fitness center where I stayed. I was not very consistent with working out at the time. It wasn't until the year 2019 when I had an eye-opening health assessment that I knew things had to change for me physically, mentally, emotionally, and psychologically. I did not want to be another statistic of my environment. So, I decided to give the one thing I hated just one more chance, and this time, I didn't regret it. For the next ten chapters, I will share with you the ten ways running has changed my outlook on life.

2

Running Boosts Weight Loss

As I started back running, I made a conscious effort to run at least 3 to 4 times a week. I set minor goals starting by running at least 1 mile each day. My goal was to shoot for 20 miles per month. After changing up my diet by cutting back on fast food, giving up a lot of sugar, eating more vegetables, and drinking more water each day, I began to see some results with the number of calories I was burning off each day from running. As I started counting calories, I noticed I was burning more calories than I was taking in at times. Within a matter of 3 months, I had gone from over 225 lbs to 190 lbs. I could tell it was working once I started getting reactions from people who knew my previous size. I then started to challenge myself even more by adding on more miles. I started trying to do 2 miles per day for 3 days a week. I would run 2 days in a row, rest the next, and run again the following day. I would then follow that up with some additional strength training.

Next, I took it a step further, I started to include high-intensity running into my workouts each week. I would do this by running fartleks, alternating between bursts of sprints and slow recovery jogs. I used the 5,4,3,2,1 method, where I would sprint for 30 seconds, followed by a slow recovery jog for 30 seconds for 5 intervals. It was very challenging yet very rewarding. I also incorporated running hills as part of my high-intensity workouts. A great benefit of high-intensity running is that you will continue to burn calories hours after your workout is complete, which is called "the after-burn effect." Also, another great benefit of high-intensity running is that it will curb your appetite, causing you to eat less, and help you to lose more weight.

We all know that carrying excessive belly fat is detrimental to our health, which increases our risk of many diseases. These high-intensity runs directly target belly fat. Just adding these two workouts to my weekly runs was a total game-changer! It allowed me to have an occasional cheat day and not have to give up some of my favorite foods. At this point, I had a better understanding of my body and what it needed.

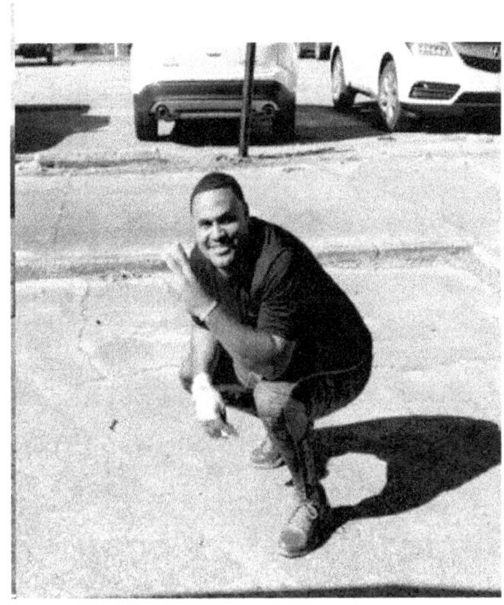
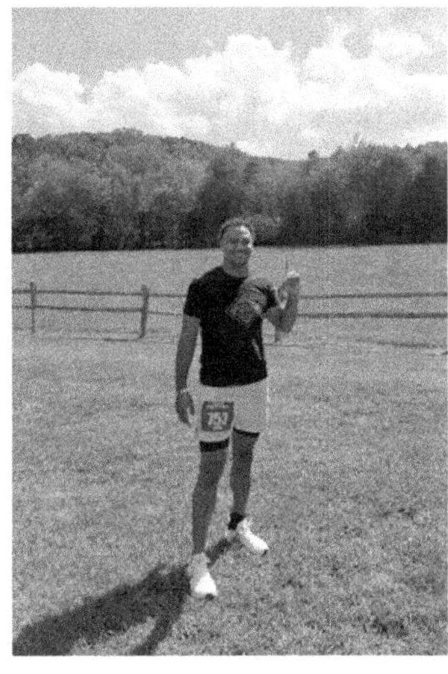

Pictured to the left weighing 225 lbs, and over to the right weighing 185 lbs

3

Running Relieves Stress and Anxiety

I often found myself not knowing who or where to turn to for guidance, when it came to dealing with stressful issues at work, sudden tragic losses, relationships, and family emergencies. I would just bottle it all up and hold it in. As I started to run daily, I began to notice this sense of peace over me. I normally would run while listening to music. Then, it was this one day I forgot to bring my headphones with me on a run, and instead of going back to get them, I decided to run without them. I turned out to enjoy it more than I expected. Just listening to Mother Nature as I ran was now my meditation. As I ran, the feeling of the wind blowing, birds chirping, grass waving, and trees swaying back and forth was very soothing to the mind. At that point, I begin to forget about all of life's issues. This was the beginning of something special.

Running had then become a part of me. If I ever started to sense a feeling of depression or anxiety building up, I now had an answer for it. The feeling I get after the run is priceless. Running releases these feel-good endorphins that will take your mind off worrying. I even noticed my mood would be different after a great run. Whatever may have upset me, was now the least of my worry. Also, I started to notice that any physical pains I had, would quickly go away due to the release of endorphins since they act as a natural painkiller.

Many people in the world today deal with stress and anxiety and are likely to be put on medication to help cope with it. This can sometimes lead to other issues due to the underlying side effects of medication. However, studies have shown that running daily can be a much better alternative with no side effects. Cortisol is a hormone that is released when you are stressed and causes many of the symptoms that come with anxiety, such as nervousness, sweating, fear, and restlessness. Going on a daily run can help burn off excess cortisol, causing less anxiety symptoms. It's such a wonderful feeling to feel relaxed and be in such a great mood. Most runners would call this the runner's high. Once you experience it, you just can't seem to get enough.

Many people suffer from loneliness which can also lead to stress. There is nothing better than getting to know yourself and what you can accomplish. If you ever feel alone, running can be a great way to feel that void and improve your mental health. This gives you time to let things slow down in your head to adjust and recharge your brain to have a positive perspective. When I'm all alone running, I never really notice it, because I'm always surrounded by God's creations. So, the next time stress and anxiety tap you on the shoulder, just grab a pair of your favorite running shoes and hit the pavement running.

4

Running Helps Build Friendships

I have competed in numerous races over the past few years, and I can say I have met some nice people through running. Some of my closest friends today, I have met from running. It is such a great feeling to meet someone that you can relate to and who shares the same love and passion for running. Running has been a great networking tool as well, which has given me the ability to meet people who work in various career fields. For example, just building strong relationships while running can sometimes lead to new job opportunities. Some of my closest friends I have met through running are financial advisors, real estate agents, professors, doctors, coaches, and the list goes on. Sometimes, some of the toughest issues you are faced with can be answered by one of your running buddies and vice versa. When you have competed in as many races as I have, you start to see a lot of the same faces during each race and you both begin to see each other's level of commitment to running. You begin to share small conversations that linger for a lifetime.

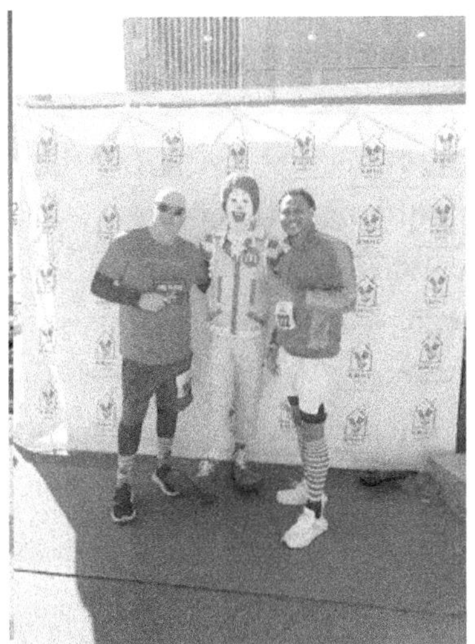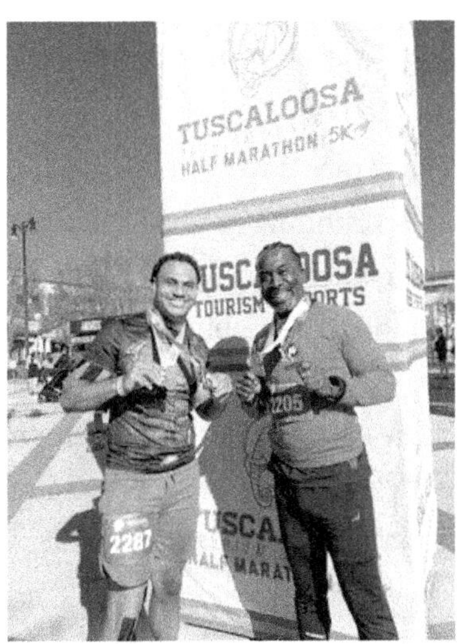

Pictured with running buddies I made over the years

Last year during one of my half-marathon races, I met a guy from South Carolina, who had driven down with his girlfriend to participate in the race. During the race, we both shared some encouraging words as we took turns passing each other along the way. After completing the race, we ended up running into each other and later sat down to talk a bit. His girlfriend, who is also a runner, competed in the race as well. After he introduced me, he later began to tell me how they met each other. He said that every time he participated in a race, he happened to run into her. She would make small talk with him each time they met. Even though they both stayed in different states, they managed to start meeting up by signing up for races competing together. She later joined our conversation to further tell the story of how they met. It was such a beautiful thing to see, two people who share the same love and passion for running brought together by that same love and passion. We later exchanged phone numbers to stay in contact and share our upcoming runs and so forth. Just like that, I met another lifelong running buddy.

I have met lots of friends who are members of running groups. One thing about running groups is that you will be with a bunch of people who will always keep you uplifted and encouraged. Whether you're an introverted person or not, building friendships through running helps improve your social skills. There is no pressure to converse when you both share the same passion. Through running, I now find it easy to walk up and spark a conversation with a total stranger. Next thing you know, we're laughing and find out we have more in common than we thought.

One of the many things I love about running is that it brings people from all walks of life together. Everyone is so encouraging. I remember a time I was battling to finish the last few miles of a half-marathon, when all of a sudden, a guy I met near the end of the race began to give me some words of encouragement and pushed me to keep going. Those words lit a fire under me to the finish line. When you build friendships through running, you always have a second option when it comes to dealing with the stresses of life. When you all meet up, you can run and talk it out at the same time. You see, running has plenty of advantages from a social standpoint.

5

Running Helps Build Discipline

As a runner, you have those days when you just want to rest and not go for a run. Those are the days when you have to dig deep and search within yourself. It's not always easy, but when you continue to push yourself, you begin to grow mentally, physically, and psychologically. The habits you make begin to shape the person you are. When you build that certain level of discipline, it makes you appreciate the smaller things, such as taking the time to make your bed every morning, washing dishes, and cleaning the house. I appreciate what running has given me from a disciplinary standpoint. Whether it's raining, hot, cold, or whatever else the condition may be, I have built up a level of mental toughness that pushes me to keep going despite of. Committing to go on a daily run takes a lot of discipline. After you have run those 3 or however many miles, your mind starts to second guess itself on the next day if you should go again or not. This is when the discipline kicks in to keep your commitment. There have been days where I have run in the rain. At this point, it was just water to me and it only made me more mentally and physically tougher.

A lot of people will never know about that extra 100% you have in you when you have reached the level of exhaustion. It's truly a beautiful thing to tap into it. Every day, my mind and body are always arguing with each other. Below is how the conversation goes most of the time.

Mind: Hello Body! I am going to run this evening when I get off work.

Body: But didn't we just run like 6 miles' yesterday?

Mind: Yes, and we are about to run 6 more. So, be ready to lace them up again this evening.

Body: I don't feel like running today. Let's just rest and get after it tomorrow.

Mind: Negative! That's not the agreement we signed up for. We have to grind on the days we feel like going and grind harder on the days we don't feel like going.

Body: OK! OK! You win! I'll be ready to go this evening. I hate you!

The way I stay consistent is by setting strict weekly goals. If you tell yourself you are going to run 20 miles in a week, you can create a plan to complete it within 4 or 5 days, but for someone who is just starting and trying to commit to running, I would say shoot for at least 10 miles a week and stick with it. You should be able to easily accomplish this within 5 days or even better, within 4 days to give yourself a free day. I am a big fan of the words "One More." I believe we all have one more in us when we are pushed to the brink, whether it be one more rep, more lap, or one more mile. To keep my level of discipline, whenever I go out for a run, I always set a goal for that day, and when I reach it, I normally counter it by adding more. For instance, I will go out to do 5 miles, and it normally turns into 6 or maybe 7. Running is a continuous thing and we must treat it as such.

6

Running Boosts The Immune System

I am living proof that running does help boost your immune system. I can't remember the last time I have ever taken a flu shot, over-the-counter medication for the common cold, or had cough drops. I run in the cold a lot as another way of building mental toughness and never have I come down with a cold from doing such. Scientifically, there are minimal amounts of immune cells that circulate throughout the body regularly. As you increase blood flow and lymph through running, you increase the movement of more immune cells from lymph nodes and the spleen into the bloodstream. After completing a run, these immune cells tend to linger around for a few hours to safeguard you from any bacteria or viruses and prevent you from becoming sick. So, if you ever wondered why you consistently are coming down with the flu or the common cold during the so-called flu season, you may want to consider going on a daily run to increase blood flow, which in turn wakes up those immune cells.

As you run for several minutes, you will notice that your body temperature gets fairly warm and later breaks into a sweat. The feeling normally carries over for a few minutes after you have completed your run. This sudden temperature rise may prevent the growth of bacteria as well as any infections. When I realized the amazing effects running had on my immune system, I never looked at the flu the same. Running can prevent you from several doctor visits treating flu-like symptoms. If you suffer from an autoimmune disorder, just listen to your body very carefully and take heed of what it needs. Starting a daily run regimen will greatly improve your disorder. When you go out for a run on a hot sunny day, you are doing your immune system a big favor by not only increasing the movement of immune cells but also getting out there for some natural Vitamin D from direct exposure to the sun. So, do your body a favor by getting out there for a run to keep that immune system strong.

7

Running Slows Down Aging

Running by far seems to be the most effective anti-aging medicine. From participating in various 5Ks and half-marathons, I tend to notice a trend in a lot of the participants. The older they get, the faster they seem. A lot of them do not show their actual age. I have the hardest time determining what age group they belong to at first glance. It's a proven fact that running does help extend your quality of life. New studies suggest that running can reverse some effects that come from sedentary aging, causing the heart to look 30 years younger by the time we reach our 70s. I must say, since I have been running over the past few years, the older I get, the younger I seem to look and the better I feel. I have even noticed that my skin is a lot smoother, which can shave off a few years. When I am often asked my age, a lot of people are often left in disbelief. At the age of 37 now, a lot of people normally take off at least 10 years.

It's proven that increased blood circulation during running gives the skin more opportunity to get nutrients from oxygen-rich blood, and new skin cells are regenerated from better oxygenation of the skin, causing your skin to have a natural shine. What truly inspires me the most is looking at the master and grand master age groups for the men and women still actively competing in 5Ks, 10Ks, half-marathons, and full-marathons. I am always amazed at their level of endurance. The pace of these runners seems to get faster and faster as if they are aging in reverse. Every time I sign up for an actual race, the first thing I do afterward is find out how old the oldest participant is.

There is this one 5K race that I competed in about 2 years ago that sticks out to me very vividly. I met this very sweet woman named Dolores. As I completed the race, I was standing around watching as the other participants came in. I ran into her husband, who I wasn't aware of at the time. He appeared to be in his mid-to-late 70s. We started a brief conversation, and I asked him if he had someone competing in the race. He then mentioned that his wife was running. I was a bit shocked. I told him that once she finished, I would love to meet her. As she finished and met up with her husband, I walked over to introduce myself. I begin to tell her that this is why I run. "You all inspire me so much!" I asked Dolores if she didn't mind telling me her age. She then told me she was 78 years old. That's right! 78 years old! I just could not believe it. I told her that she didn't look a day over 60. Her skin was very smooth with a glow, and she showed no signs of wrinkles. What Dolores says is a testament to her longevity in running. She said she used to run lots of marathons in her younger days, and even though she doesn't do long-distance running now, she still manages to run in a lot of 5Ks. I secretly got her bib number to check her race finish time, and it was a shocking 35 minutes at 78, which is impressive! This is a great example of what can happen when you have a lifelong commitment to running. I just had to get a picture with her, because she is truly an inspiration to us all.

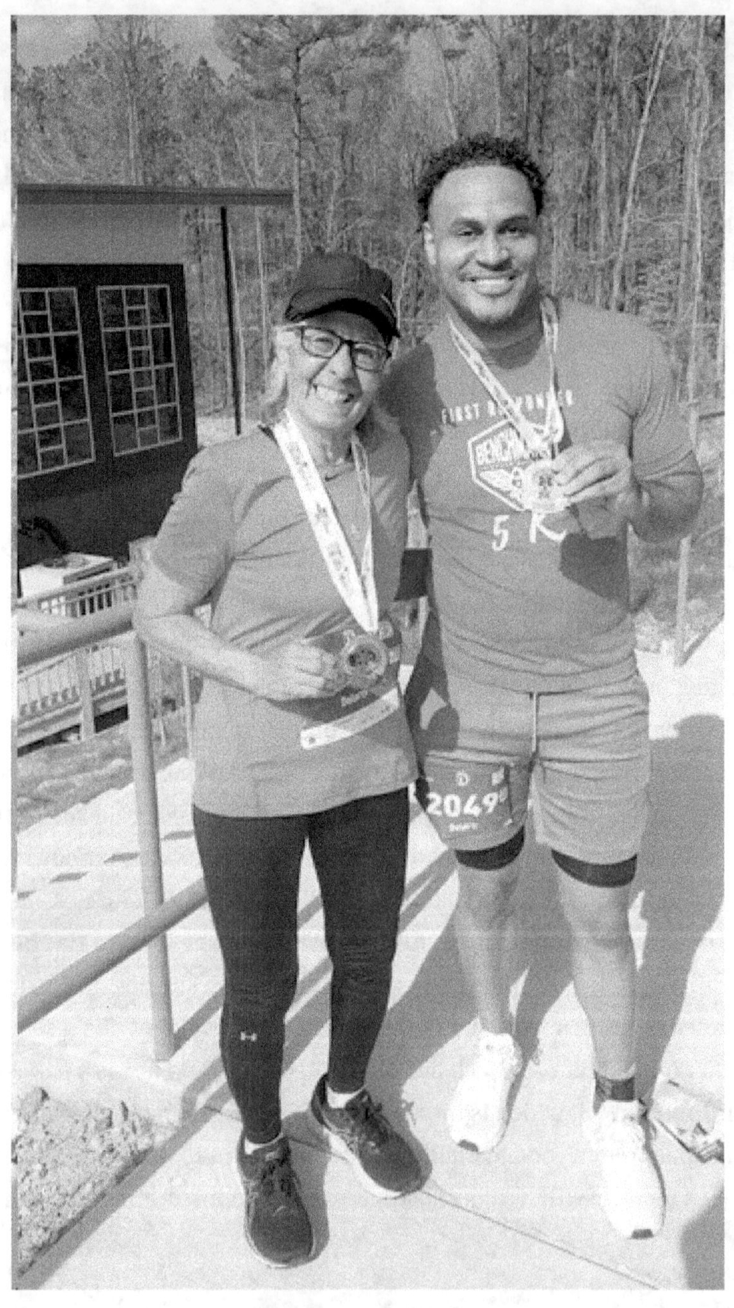

Me and Dolores after 5K race

It's never too late to take a few years off your age and bring back your skin's natural glow. Just lace up your favorite pair of running shoes and go out for a nice run. I know a lot of people tend to put themselves in a box when it comes to aging, saying what they can't do anymore, but I am here to tell you that even if you're in your mid-40s - 60s, it's still not too late to start.

8

Running Increases Your Energy

As I began my running journey, I can honestly say my energy level was fairly low. I seemed to get tired fairly quickly. I found it difficult to run 2 to 3 miles at a time without crashing, but through lots and lots of repetition, I started to see gradual improvements. The more I ran, the better it got. My breathing tremendously improved. I then started to consistently run 3 miles each day as my target goal. My run times weren't all that great, but I stuck with it. After about 2 years of running, I began to notice my speed increasing. My 5K pace was getting faster and faster. It wasn't until a friend of mine told me that I needed to start adding more miles that I realized my full capability. I was able to cover more miles without stopping. I went from running 3 miles/day to later doing 4 to 5 miles a day. Now, that has easily increased to 6 miles. Some days, I may go out and run 8 to 10 miles just to challenge myself or in training mode. I went from competing in 5Ks to competing in half-marathons.

In my wildest dreams, I never would have thought I could run over 13.2 miles non-stop. I challenged myself and competed in (3) half-marathons in the year 2023. Each time, I noticed an increase in my finishing times. I went from 2:15:45 down to 1:54:49.

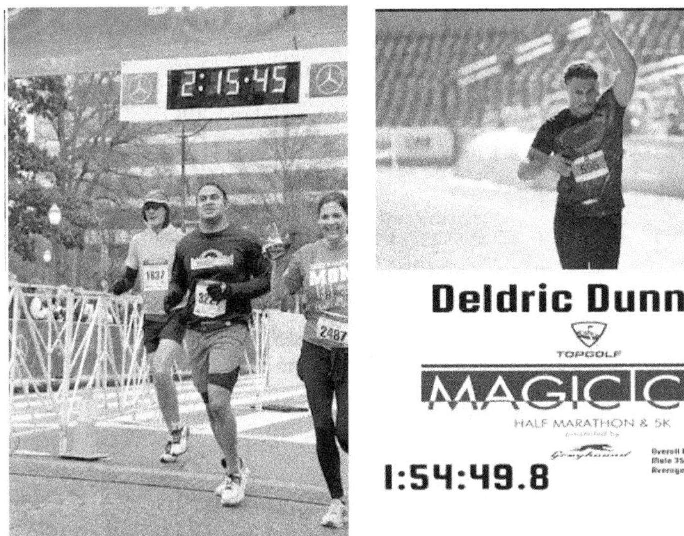

Pictured to the left was my first half-marathon and to the right was my last one for the year

My energy level had gone to an all-time high. However, if it wasn't for staying consistent, this would not have been possible. I now finish long runs with the feeling that I can do more. I no longer feel sluggish throughout the day. I know it may sound a bit weird that by moving more you can increase your energy levels when you would normally think otherwise. However, there is some pretty interesting science behind that. According to Harvard Medical, exertion causes your body to produce more mitochondria inside your muscle cells. Mitochondria, known as the powerhouse of the cells, creates fuel out of glucose from the food you eat and oxygen from the air you breathe in. Having more mitochondria increases your body's energy supply. The oxygen boosts you get from running not only support the mitochondria's energy production but also allow your body to perform a lot better.

Normally, when I begin running, I try to start at a relatively slow pace to get the blood flowing. It's normal to have a little fatigue as you start, especially if your body has been resting for a fairly long time. Listen to your body. Run at a comfortable pace until it feels relaxed and gradually pick up the pace. It's also good to change things up a bit. So, instead of going on a long slow-paced run, incorporate some sprints into your daily run routine to help build up your stamina and increase your lung capacity over time. You will begin to notice how relaxed your breathing is the longer you run. When I watch the elite runners, I always wonder how they can withstand such stamina at a rapid pace over a very long distance. Through very rigorous training over long periods doing things such as hill workouts, high-intensity sprints, and strict breathing exercises, you can strengthen the diaphragm allowing you to pace yourself much better.

I used to get discouraged during my races when I started and a lot of older runners were passing me. Yet, they didn't seem as if they were going faster than me. The reason they were is because their breathing was a lot more relaxed than mine. Paying attention to your breathing can help you determine your pace and possibly tolerate a more challenging, speedier pace. Having a run partner that is a lot faster than you can be very beneficial for optimizing energy gains. For one, you will do your best to keep up with them as you all carry on conversation. As the pace picks up, you hardly may notice it, because you are so engaged in what they are saying. The more you run with them, you will eventually notice a much faster pace. The one key element is to never stop pushing your limits.

9

Running Strengthens Bone Structure

When it comes to running, there are a lot of people who have a negative perception of it. Most will tell you that they choose not to run because it has a bad impact on your knees over time. However, research shows that running creates positive bone metabolic activity, which means that runners store a higher concentration of bone-building hormones and enzymes. This translates to increased calcium uptake by our bones, ultimately increasing bone density. Running to me is like another form of lifting weights. As you run, your arms continue to move in a forward and backward position. This continuous movement can help build more muscles in your shoulders, back, biceps, and forearms when done over a long period. Also, running helps strengthen your quadriceps, hamstrings, calves, abdomen, glutes, as well as hip flexors. Over time since I have been running, I have seen a noticeable change in my entire muscle profile. The continued stress of the muscles that are working to allow you to keep moving is constantly pulling on your bones which has an immediate effect on bone density.

Before I started running, 3 to 4 times a week, I used to experience quite a bit of knee pain. As I started to increase my running, I noticed the pain started to shift away the more I did it. From what I can tell, the bones seem to get stronger when put under the stress of high-intensity running. Running is very impact and when your foot continuously strikes the ground, it jerks and shocks the bone. Rest and recovery allow your bones plenty of time to get to work repairing and strengthening themselves. Osteoblast, which are bone cells that constantly produce new bone, is stimulated. Whereas, Osteoclast, which is constantly breaking down bone to release minerals stored inside, is reduced so that the bone is strengthened back up. It's been proven that running can have a positive impact when it comes to osteoporosis. Study shows that it reduces the rate of bone loss and conserves bone tissue, which lowers the risk of having any fractures. When I talk to older, more experienced runners, I'm always willing to take any advice they may give, and one of the main questions I tend to ask is, "Do you ever have any pain in your knees?" The rapid response I normally get is no, and their advice is to stay active. When you lead a very sedentary lifestyle, weak muscles tend to increase causing bone fractures. When I see 70 and 80-year-olds still out there running, it validates the age-old question of whether running is bad for your knees, which is just the motivation I needed to continue running.

We all know that injuries can still occur during high-intensity activities such as running. There are several tips you can take to help prevent injury when running. Always warm up before running by incorporating lots of stretching. Do at least 30 minutes of stretching before engaging in any running. Also, make sure to include stretches when you are finishing up a run. If you are going to be running daily, you also want to frequently change up your running surface. Instead of just running on the pavement, alternate between other surfaces such as dirt, grass, trail, or indoor/outdoor track to reduce the impact on your knees now and then. By doing so, you prevent the risk of lower leg injuries from overexertion. Always make sure to use the proper technique when running. For example, if you are doing a lot of heel striking, you run the risk of injury. Run within your current fitness level to avoid strains of your lower extremities. Then, you can gradually pick up the intensity. Also, make sure you have the proper running shoes on for the surface you will be running on to prevent any leg pain or blisters that could arise. There are many more tips out there, but these are some of the most important when preparing for a daily run.

10

Running Helps Promote Good Sleeping Habits

If you are not sleeping well, and finding it hard to close your eyes, here's an idea. Go for a run. For the longest, I have struggled to go to sleep getting enough rest. I always found myself up very late trying to wind down, and when I closed my eyes, it only felt like a few minutes. I wake up very sluggish and half the time, I'm not in the best of moods. Ever since I have made running a part of my daily life, my quality of sleep has greatly improved. When I complete a long run, I feel so relaxed. After a warm bath and a hot meal, I am ready to lie down. The struggle in going to bed is a thing of the past. When I wake up, I feel so well-rested. That runner's high is very contagious. It makes my decision whether or not I'm going to run for the day simple.

Once your body releases those feel-good hormones, it almost instantly relaxes the mind. According to research, running can intensify the amount of deep sleep that an individual gets. Deep sleep normally happens about 10 minutes after you fall asleep and can last from 40 to 90 minutes during the first episode and gets shorter thereafter on each rotation. When you're in a night of deep sleep or slow wave sleep, your breathing, heartbeat, body temperature, and brain waves all slow down while the body goes to work cleaning out toxins, releasing human growth hormones, and consolidating memories to help repair muscle, bone, and tissue damage. The beauty of this is that the more you run, you increase the possibility of having more deep sleep, and the longer you spend sleeping like this, the faster your recovery time will be from running pains.

A regular running routine can certainly lead to an improvement in your total sleep time as well as the time spent falling asleep. Other disorders such as sleep apnea and restless legs syndrome can be reduced by having a normal running routine. According to the Sleep Foundation, many people experience insomnia due to a misaligned internal body clock. Depending on when you go for your daily run can help to reset the body's internal clock and in turn, cause them to fall asleep sooner. Running will boost the hormone serotonin, which is involved in the sleep-wake cycle. Establishing a bedtime routine is very important if you are not getting enough sleep regularly. It can help create healthy habits that trigger the brain to get ready for bed. For starters, set a decent bedtime, get off your phone, take a nice warm bath, turn off the TV 30 minutes or so before bed, and do some light stretching to relax the body. When you wake up in the morning, I know we are all guilty of it, but try to limit hitting the snooze on that alarm clock. As you get up, go right ahead and start making up your bed. It sets the tone for the day. If you continuously follow this routine for a few weeks, it will become a part of you, just like running.

11

Running Boosts Your Confidence

Running gives me the feeling that I can accomplish anything I set my mind to do. When I go out to complete a daily run, it's a major confidence booster. Just the fact of setting a distinct number of miles, minutes, or laps to run, and not only completing it but adding more, prepares you for any challenges you face in a race. As I am training for a race, I always prepare for the worst. I try to put myself in the most uncomfortable position possible so that I am that much more confident that there is nothing that will affect me on the course. Most race courses tend to be very hilly. So, instead of just running on a surface with little elevation, I will go and find running routes that have lots of hills and add a few extra miles. Tackling my planned workout gives me the ultimate confidence that when race time comes around, I will be prepared. If I'm running a race, and I know it is going to be hot, I would make a plan to train in the hottest part of the day and add on some hills along the way to make it uncomfortable. The same applies to those winter months. When you are consistent with the process, you will easily adapt to your environment.

I have competed in races in just about every weather condition except snow. I do those uncomfortable runs, because it will mentally, physically, and psychologically prepare your mind for what's ahead. So, if the weather forecast says that there is going to be a 50% chance of rain all week leading up to the race, guess what? I'll be outside in the rain running. That way, you are not worried about the conditions anymore. Your only goal is to finish because you have put in the work. About 2 years ago, I competed in a 5K cave run. The whole week leading up to the race, it was raining non-stop. I had previously done the run before but I was not physically prepared for what was ahead of me. This route had by far the highest elevation I had ever run before. It was roughly over 800 ft. by the time I reached the finish line. It kicked my butt! However, the next time around, I knew what to look for and how to train. As I mentioned earlier, it was raining the entire week. So, I set out to do a few runs in the rain leading up to the race. I made sure to add some hill workouts along the way. Also, I always added extra miles to complete each workout run. After consistently completing those workouts, and noticing my pace was getting faster, I was more than confident on race day, no matter the condition. As it came time for the race, it was great weather outside. The sun was out, but there was a small chance of rain. About 1.5 miles into the race, it began to storm. I started smiling because this was what I prepared for. I crushed my finishing time from the previous year.

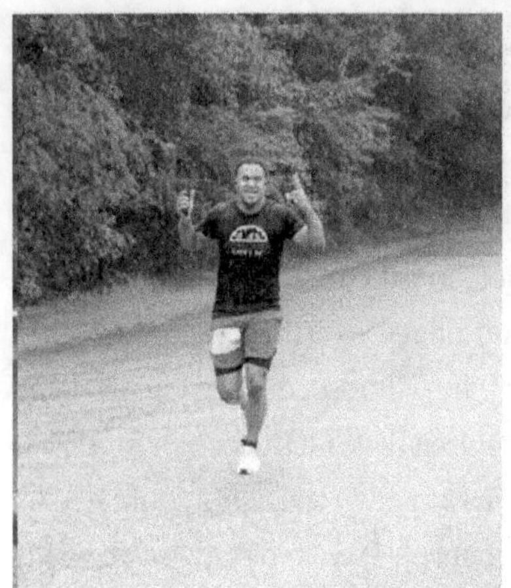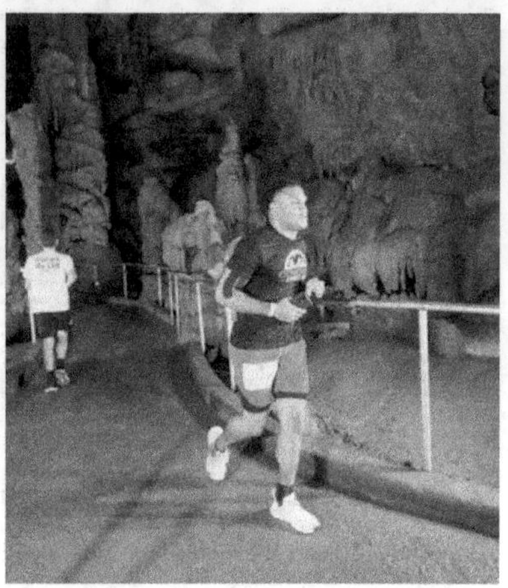

2022 5K Cave Run Pictured to the left is me running in the rain and to the right is me now inside the cave

When you start to see the many health benefits of running such as weight loss, normal blood pressure and blood sugar ranges, a strong immune system, and much better sleep, you start to feel very confident about yourself, which gets addictive. Running greatly improves your cognitive function by providing the brain with important nutrients and oxygen. When you are done with your workout, you leave with the feeling that you can tackle any task put in front of you, as well as improve your self-esteem. At some point in our lives, we all in some way have negatively talked down on ourselves. You can easily turn that negative into a positive by getting in a run. People may say I'm crazy, but I have frequent conversations with myself, especially on runs. I could be coming up on my last mile, after telling myself to do one more and completing it, that extra mile goes a very long way. You leave the workout with your self-esteem running very high. It sounds crazy, but you start to think differently. Your food choices may change. After a successful run, instead of fast food, you may decide to get a healthy salad and a bottle of water. The reason I'm saying this is because I tend to do it a lot. A lot of the foods I used to crave, I don't have a taste for. I have gradually changed the way I think about food and what goes in my body, all because of a simple run. Give it a try. In due time, you will see exactly what I am talking about. I love being around my running community. They are some of the most positive and uplifting people to be around. Their energy is contagious, which can easily boost your self-esteem.

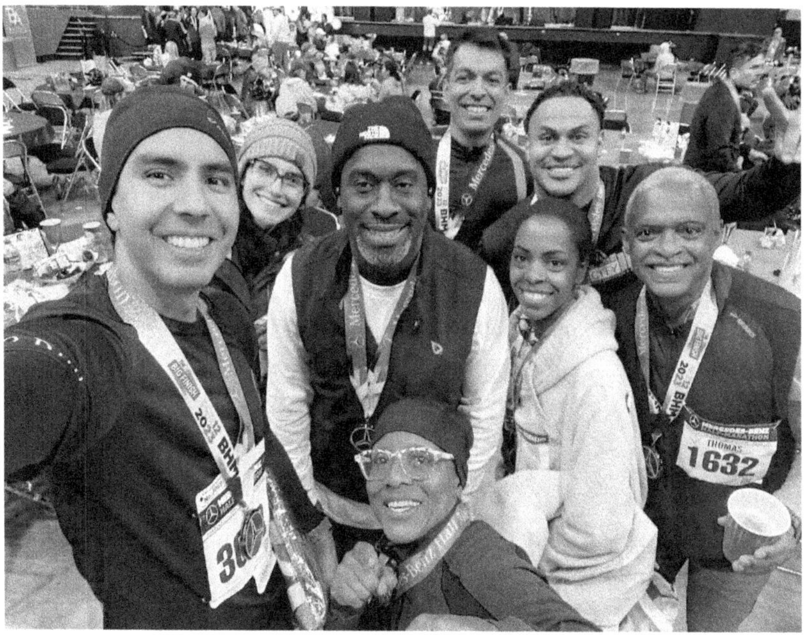

2023 Mercedez-Benz Half-Marathon Pictured with running friends after completing my first-ever half-marathon

12

Conclusion

In conclusion, running, as you can see, has opened up a whole new world for me. My outlook on life these days is very different. Running has transformed my life completely. My entire thought process is different. My confidence is through the roof. My energy level is at an all-time high, now that I am at a healthier weight. I feel like I can run for days. Due to an enhanced immune system, I don't worry as much as I once did about coming down with a cold or flu. I am more socially engaged than ever before. I no longer have to deal with any stress and anxiety. If you ever start to feel any symptoms of stress, you should be well prepared on how to cope with it. From a disciplinary standpoint, I stay focused on my daily tasks and never let anything get in the way of it. If I ever need some positive reinforcement, I can always reach out to my running community. I am aging gracefully by living a better lifestyle and you too can reap all the same benefits by embarking on the journey of running. If you are tired of the way you look or feel, I challenge you to put on a pair of running shoes and go outside for a brisk run. Try it and you just might love it. Please be sure to leave a review if you enjoyed this book.

13

Resources

1. OpenAI. (n.d.). Home - OpenAI. https://www.openai.com/

2. Healthline. (n.d.). Running for Weight Loss: 6 Tips for Success. Retrieved from https://www.healthline.com/nutrition/running-for-weight-loss#TOC_TITLE_HDR_4

3. Gundersen Health System. (n.d.). Exercise and Your Immune System. Retrieved from https://www.gundersenhealth.org/health-wellness/move/exercise-and-your-immune-system#:~:text=Not%20only%20does%20exercise%20get,keep%20you%20from%20getting%20sick.

4. Calm Clinic. (n.d.). 3 Things to Try if You Feel Anxious About Running. Retrieved from https://www.calmclinic.com/anxiety/3-things-to-try

5. MedlinePlus. (n.d.). Exercise and Immunity. Retrieved from https://medlineplus.gov/ency/article/007165.htm#:~:text=Physical%20activity%20may%20help%20flush,system%20cells%20that%20fight%20disease.

6. Fleet Feet. (n.d.). How Running Makes Your Body Younger. Re-

trieved from https://www.fleetfeet.com/blog/how-running-makes-your-body-younger#:~:text=While%20we%20can't%20stay,time%20we%20reach%20our%2070s.

7. Harvard Health Publishing. (n.d.). Does Exercise Really Boost Energy Levels? Retrieved from https://www.health.harvard.edu/exercise-and-fitness/does-exercise-really-boost-energy-levels

8. Kerlan-Jobe Orthopaedic Clinic. (n.d.). Running Your Way to Better Bone and Brain Health. Retrieved from https://kerlanjobe.org/running-your-way-to-better-bone-and-brain-health/#:~:text=Running%20creates%20favorable%20bone%20metabolic,which%20ultimately%20increases%20bone%20density.

9. Better Health Channel. (n.d.). Osteoporosis and Exercise. Retrieved from https://www.betterhealth.vic.gov.au/health/conditionsandtreatments/osteoporosis-and-exercise

10. Dr. Juliet McGrattan. (2023, January 25). How Does Running Help Bone Strength? Retrieved from https://drjulietmcgrattan.com/2023/01/25/how-does-running-help-bone-strength/

11. Spartan. (n.d.). Is Running Good for Sleep? Retrieved from https://www.spartan.com/blogs/unbreakable-focus/is-running-good-for-sleep

12. Sleep Foundation. (n.d.). Exercise and Insomnia. Retrieved from https://www.sleepfoundation.org/insomnia/exercise-and-insomnia#:~:text=Exercise%20may%20realign%20your%20internal%20body%20clock.&text=Further%2C%20some%20forms%20of%20exercise,metabolize%20serotonin%20and%20regulate%20sleep